THE PEACEFUL EATING PLANNER

90 DAYS OF JOURNAL PROMPTS AND COACHING EXERCISES
FOR MAKING PEACE WITH FOOD

Karen Lynne Oliver, BA, MA
Founder of *Beyond the Bathroom Scale*®

Copyright © 2020 by Karen Lynne Oliver

All rights reserved. No part of this publication may be reproduced, distributed, or transmitted in any form or by any means, including photocopying, recording, or other electronic or mechanical methods, without the prior written permission of the author, except in the case of brief quotations embodied in critical reviews and certain other non-commercial uses, permitted by copyright law.

For permission requests, please email the author via the address below:

karenoliver@beyondthebathroomscale.co.uk

"*Beyond the Bathroom Scale*" is a Registered UK Trademark and the intellectual property of Karen Lynne Oliver, trading as *Beyond the Bathroom Scale®*, part of Lynne Media ('our', 'we', 'us').

We take the protection of our intellectual property very seriously. If we discover that you have breached the terms of the licence, we may bring legal proceedings against you and seek monetary damages and/or an injunction to stop you using our materials. You could also be ordered to pay our legal costs.

ISBN: 9798651120994

Imprint: Independently published for Lynne Media

Cover Image: Canva

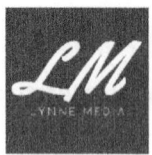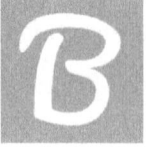

LEGAL DISCLAIMER

By continuing to use this planner you acknowledge and agree to the full disclaimer.

This planner is not appropriate for people with active eating disorders; if you are suffering from an eating disorder or have suffered from one in the past please seek professional advice from your GP instead.

Although this planner is intended to help heal your body image, it may be triggering for anyone who has an underlying eating disorder or illness such as body dysmorphia.

For Educational and Informational Purposes Only

The information provided in or through this Website is for educational and informational purposes only and solely as a self-help tool for your own use.

Not a Substitute for Professional Advice

I am not a registered therapist, dietitian, personal trainer, or any other kind of health professional and do not hold myself out to be. The information contained in this Website is not intended to be a substitute for health or wellbeing advice that can be provided by your own GP or health and wellbeing practitioner. The advice found on this Website should be treated as a suggestion, based on my own personal experience of what works for me, rather than from medical training. This programme is not a substitute for seeking professional help with eating disorders or other mental health issues.

Although care has been taken in preparing the information provided to you, I cannot be held responsible for any errors or omissions, and I accept no liability whatsoever for any loss or damage you may incur. Always seek health care advice from a registered professional, relating to your specific circumstances as needed for all questions and concerns you now have, or may have in the future. You agree that the information in this planner and on the website is not professional health care advice.

For everyone who has felt at war with food their whole lives.

It's time to end the fight.

The Peaceful Eating Planner

ABOUT THE AUTHOR

Karen Lynne Oliver, BA, MA, is the founder of *Beyond the Bathroom Scale®*, a hub of self-help resources to aid with recovery from disordered eating and body image.

Beyond the Bathroom Scale® was awarded 'Most Innovative Digital Health Business, UK' in 2020 by Acquisition International.

A former Social Worker, Karen holds a bachelor's degree in Sociology, specialising in health and society and a master's degree in Social Work. She has trained in counselling skills and psychotherapy-based approaches including Cognitive Behavioural Therapy (CBT), Dialectical Behavioural Therapy (DBT) and Motivational Interviewing (MI).

Karen has previously written for *HuffPost UK* and has been featured in *The Metro, Calm Moment, The Cambridge Independent* and *Cosmopolitan Magazine*.

FREE RESOURCES

Over on *Beyond the Bathroom Scale*® you can sign up to a **free six-day course** which includes 6 video lessons, a PDF workbook, and a guide to recommended resources.

The free six-day course covers:

1. What we mean by diet culture, how to recognise it, why it's harmful to your health and how to rebel against it.

2. Why self-compassion and body acceptance is essential for health.

3. How to listen to what your body is trying to tell you it needs most.

4. The causes behind emotional eating and the strategies for tackling it.

5. What is meant by Intuitive Eating and how it can help you gain freedom from dieting and improve your relationship with food and your body.

6. What the Health at Every Size® (HAES) movement is all about and the body of research which supports taking an anti-diet approach to improving physical health.

You can sign up for free and get started straight away using this link:

https://www.beyondthebathroomscale.co.uk/health-mindset-starter-kit

USEFUL LINKS:

- **[FREE] The Health Mindset Starter Kit:**
  https://www.beyondthebathroomscale.co.uk/health-mindset-starter-kit

- **[FREE] BTBS Community Support Facebook Group:**
  https://www.facebook.com/groups/btbsblog/

- **The Health Mindset Programme™:**
  https://www.beyondthebathroomscale.co.uk/thehealthmindsetprogramme/

- **Facebook Page:**
  https://www.facebook.com/BeyondTheBathroomScale/

- **Instagram:**
  https://www.instagram.com/beyondthebathroomscale

HOW TO USE THIS PLANNER

The Peaceful Eating Planner for people who want to leave diets behind once and for all and embrace Intuitive and mindful eating instead.

The workbook is split into three parts:

1. Developing Body Awareness - check in with your body's signals, including your hunger and fullness cues.
2. Unconditional Permission to Eat – understand and ditch the food rules you've adopted from past diets and diet culture.
3. Mindful Eating – find enjoyment and satisfaction from food and listen out for pesky thoughts of diets creeping back into your mind.

If you'd like to know more about the anti-diet approach, intuitive eating and cognitive behavioural therapy, please visit my website at **https://www.beyondthebathroomscale.co.uk** and sign up for the **FREE 6-day course** on making peace with food and body.

Each section of this planner starts with coaching exercises and has 30 days of daily planner pages tailored to the goals of each of the three section. The daily planner pages also have sections for recording your mood and gratitude journaling.

Logging your mood can be useful for highlighting the link between your body image and your mood. For example, when we're happy about something, we may be less focused on our bodies. Likewise, our body image can impact our mood, so we may feel sad, anxious, or withdrawn on days where we feel low about our bodies.

A daily gratitude practice can help interrupt the seemingly never-ending stream of anxious thinking we can find ourselves trapped in when our stress levels are too high (known as ruminating). The simple act of taking one minute each day to write down three things you are grateful for (even small things like the weather, or someone letting you out of a busy junction) can really improve your mood by helping to put negative events into perspective and reminding you that life does have beauty in it, even in depths of the toughest of times.

WHAT DO WE MEAN BY EATING INTUITIVELY?

Peaceful eating means you're able to eat without feelings of anxiety or guilt. You have no food rules, you do not diet, and you eat the foods which make you feel good and satisfy you.

Intuitive eating is big part of this. When we eat according to our intuition, we're letting our body's signals guide us on when we eat, how much we eat, and what we eat. We also don't adhere to food rules or diet plans and instead give ourselves unconditional permission to eat. We all start our lives knowing how to eat intuitively.

We can see young toddlers demonstrate intuitive eating every time they ask for food, push their plate away, or pick and poke at different foods on their plate, inspecting them intently. Young toddlers eat mindfully, refuse to eat past the point of fullness and will certainly let you know about it when they're hungry!

WHAT RUINED OUR RELATIONSHIP WITH FOOD?

You may be wondering, why and when did we lose this ability? The trouble is, in modern day western society, there are many factors in the average adult's life that disrupts our intuition.

Such as:

- **DIET CULTURE** - Diet culture causes us to lose trust in our bodies by telling us that we're out of control around food and need to restrict intake and follow a diet plan. It positions other people as the experts on our bodies, rather than ourselves. Diet culture prioritizes weight loss over health, and this is often reflected in our eating habits, such as opting for the lowest calorie or so-called 'healthy foods, at the cost of our satisfaction for the sake of weight loss. This causes us to feel deprived or punished and can later lead to binge eating. With so much conflicting nutritional research around we also feel confused about what we 'should be eating'.

- **HECTIC LIFESTYLES** - Our hectic modern lives make it challenging to meet our hunger cues when we first notice them. This often results in us becoming ravenous by the time we do get time to eat and therefore increases the risk of binge eating.

- **FOOD OBSESSED SOCIETY** - Our social lives revolve around food; adverts for food are everywhere and restaurants are always promoting offers, big plate specials and buy one get one free. This can make us feel like we need more food than we do. Food marketeers know exactly what psychological cues triggers our ear, nose and eye hunger and they spend tonnes of cash exploiting this, from the carefully crafted written descriptions and photographs on menus, to the smell of a bakery down the road, and even the lighting and colours used in a restaurant's interior.

- **REACTING TO EMOTIONS** - Elements of our culture teaches us to soothe ourselves with food and drink – "treat yourself to a slice of cake, you deserve it", "unwind after a hard day with a glass of wine". This can also be learned in childhood, for example, if you were given chocolate to stop you crying or rewarded with sweets. Sometimes we're afraid to 'feel' strong emotions, because of our beliefs about emotions, and look for a means to 'numb' or distract ourselves from them. Because food is enjoyable and readily available, it's seen as a reliable source of comfort and pleasure for us, and so begins the habit of emotional eating.

IN A DIFFERENT WORLD...

In other words, if we lived in a cultural vacuum, with no concept of diets, no ideals about body shape and weight, no marketing of foods and the practice of mindfulness and self-reflection when it came to emotions, we would all be intuitive eaters.

INITIAL EXERCISES

Imagine eating food without a side of guilt and shame

PEACEFUL EATING SELF-ASSESSMENT

To begin, let's run through a quick exercise to get some idea of the scale of your body awareness and intuitive eating. Read through the statements below and tick the ones you agree with or feel apply to you most of the time.

I avoid certain foods groups or ingredients (which I do not have an allergy or intolerance to) because I believe that cutting these foods out will help with weight loss. (e.g. carbs, grains, gluten, dairy).	
I permit myself to have 'cheat days' or 'cheat meals', where I allow myself to eat whatever I want.	
If I want to eat something I view as 'extra' in a day, like a dessert, I feel like I need to exercise more, i.e. the 'burn it to earn it' philosophy.	
If I know I'm going out for a meal with friends in the evening, I cut back on food in the day to account for it.	
I carefully eat all week, and then eat whatever I want at the weekends, regardless of how hungry or full I feel.	
I count and track calories.	

I try to adhere to a calorie or points/Syns goal most days, regardless of how hungry or full I am.	
If I eat 'forbidden' foods ('treats', 'junk' or 'bad'), I feel like I've blown it and then experience the 'f*ck it effect', where I eat everything in large quantities and ignore my hunger/fullness cues.	
If I feel like I ate too much at one meal, I deliberately eat less at the next to 'make up for it', regardless of how hungry I am.	
I describe my day of food as either 'good' or 'bad'.	
I say things like "getting back on plan" or "falling off the wagon".	
I eat foods I don't like because I consider them 'healthy'.	
I have a list of foods I consider 'bad' or 'forbidden'.	
I refer to some foods as 'guilt free'.	
When I feel hungry, I look for ways to distract myself from the urge to eat.	

I feel the need to clear my plate, regardless of how full I feel.	
I struggle to recognise fullness long before I feel uncomfortably full	
I have difficulty judging how much to eat.	
I have difficulty deciding what I should eat.	
I decide what and how much to eat based on my calorie (or points/Syns) goal for the day, regardless of how hungry I'm feeling.	

Tally up the number of ticks and make a note of your score below. We'll repeat this self-assessment again at the end of the planner to see how far you've progressed. The lower the score, the better.

Today's date	
My score	

SECTION 1: DEVELOPING BODY AWARENESS

Your body has many ways of communicating its needs to you, but you must learn its language and listen

WHAT IS BODY AWARENESS?

Body awareness is the ability to pick up on your body's signals and understand the meaning of them. If you are truly on a mission to make peace with food and your body, you will need to develop this awareness so that you can listen in to your body's cues and effectively meet its needs. Whether it is about getting more sleep, changing up eating habits, swapping to a relaxing form of exercise, or even addressing a negative relationship in your life which is tearing you down emotionally.

WHY IS THIS IMPORTANT FOR YOUR HEALTH?

An essential part of intuitive eating (an alternative to dieting, which we will go into more depth in the next section) is an awareness of hunger, fullness, and satiety. Therefore, it's important that you develop the skill of mindfully watching out for your bodies cues and get into the habit of remembering to mentally check in with yourself before, during and after eating, or that you can eat accordingly.

As for overcoming emotional eating, an awareness of our thought patterns and feelings is crucial in order to identify, correctly label, and work through our emotions, rather than attempt to distract from or numb them with food (which I cover in *The Emotional Eating Workbook Planner*).

With these two aims in mind, let's look at some examples of cues you will benefit from becoming mindful of.

EXAMPLES OF BODY CUES TO LOOK OUT FOR

When there's a need going unmet, you can be sure that your body will let you know about it, but it may not always be so straightforward or easy to pick up.

A really good book written by a doctor on the topic of body awareness, or 'body intelligence' is *Body Wise*, by Dr Rachel Carlton Abrams (Bluebird, 2017). In this book, Dr Carlton Abrams describes a wide range of strange symptoms experienced by her patients which were treated by resolving seemingly un-related issues in their lives.

Aside from illness and pain, other cues to listen out for (or in many cases, learn to recognise) are:

- Physical hunger - the kind you feel in your stomach, not your mouth or your mind

- Feelings of fullness and satiety

- Thirst - which is often mistaken for hunger

- Tiredness - sometimes confused for a lack of motivation and focus

- Emotional distress - which can often lead to emotional eating, whereby individuals eat for the sole purpose of making themselves 'feel' better emotionally, for example, comfort eating after a stressful day at work.

- Tension in the body - for example, tension or a feeling of tightness or heaviness in the shoulders can be a sign of stress.

PERFORMING A BODY SCAN

In this exercise you are going to relax, get comfortable and take 10 minutes out of our day to run through what is referred to as a 'body scan'. This is where we'll tune out from the outside world for a short time, and fully focus on the sensations going through our body, such as our breathing, our heart rate and how tense or relaxed each part of our body feels.

It's a basic meditation exercise and it's incredibly useful for helping you press pause on the day and really check in with yourself and your body's cues- whether you choose to do this while sitting at your desk on a lunch break, in bed first thing in the morning before getting up or even sitting eyes open on the bus home from work!

To begin with I want you to find a place you can sit comfortably with a straight back and feet on the floor or lie down flat if you prefer. Make sure you will not be disturbed while you are practicing this exercise - and please put your phone on do not disturb. Please do not listen to this track while driving or engaged in any other activity.

For the next few minutes, I just want you to focus on your body and tune out from the outside world.

- Begin by taking a deep breath in through your nose, and out though the mouth. Take another deep breath in through your nose. And out through your mouth. Breathing relaxation in through your nose and breathing tension out through your mouth. Deep breath in.... And slowly exhale. Slowly inhale....... softly exhale.
- As you continue to breathe deeply, I want you to focus on the physical sensation of the surface you are resting on.

- Is it firm or soft? Cold or warm? Which parts of your body have contact with the surface you are resting on?
- Take a few moments to scan down through the body, and as you do this, I want you to examine how each part of your body is feeling. Starting with your face, I want you think about whether you are holding any tension in your facial muscles. Relax your eyes. Relax your jaw. Relax your neck. Relax your shoulders.
- Move down towards your arms, noticing any tension and relaxing each part as we go. Your hands. Your fingers.
- Take a moment to notice where you are breathing from. As you inhale, does your chest rise? Or your stomach? If you struggle to tell, you can place your hands just below your chest to increase an awareness of your breath.
- Can you hear or feel the rate of your heartbeat? Not everyone can straight away, but the more you do this exercise, the more conscious you will become of your body's cues.
- Move your attention down to your lower body. Relax your hips, the muscles in your bottom and thighs. Release any tension in your calves. And let your feet and toes relax.
- Notice how you are feeling. What sort of mood are you in right now?
- Now take your attention back to the breath.
- Return to where you feel the rising and falling sensation of the breath most strongly. Notice how each breath feels. Are they long or short breaths? Deep or shallow? Rough or smooth?
- Begin to count the breaths as you focus on the rising and falling sensation, count 1 with the rise and 2 with the fall, continuing to do this until you reach the count of 10.
- Now I want you to let go of any focus and let your mind do whatever it wants to for a few moments.
- Bring the mind back to the sensation of the surface you are resting on and notice which parts of your body are in contact with it.

Well done for completing your first body scan. I now want you to take a moment to jot down some thoughts about how you found the exercise.
- Do you feel calmer?
- Did you notice any physical tension or sensations in your body during the exercise?
- Could you pick up on your heart rate?

Jot some thoughts down before we move onto the exercise.

RECOGNISING HUNGER

A pivotal aspect of Intuitive Eating is developing (or rather re-learning) the ability to identify whether you are physically hungry, and then meeting that need unconditionally. I want to emphasise that this is not about reducing Intuitive Eating down to the soundbite of "only eat when you are physically hungry", Intuitive eating is much more than that! Having a truly peaceful relationship with food means also having a non-judgemental awareness of the different *types* of hunger we experience, such as emotional hunger or hunger triggered by our senses, rather than a physical hunger or biological urge for nourishment.

Sometimes we will turn to food for enjoyment or comfort at a time when we're not experiencing physical (stomach) hunger, or we'll eat something simply because it stimulates our senses; a food looks, sounds and smells delicious, and so we want it! All of this is a perfectly normal part of the human existence and isn't something to feel guilty about (as the diet industry would have you believe).

SYMPTOMS OF BIOLOGICAL HUNGER

To make sure that we always meet our physical need for hunger, we need to have an awareness of what biological (physical) hunger feels like.

As you read this next section, I want you to think about how aware you are when you experience these sensations and what actions you take.

- Do you dismiss them?
- Do you mistake them for something else?
- Or do you leave it too long to meet them and then feel the urge to binge eat when you finally come to eat?

I also want to note that we're all different and there's no one way to feel biological hunger - you may not experience all these sensations, you may even experience sensations I haven't listed here.

Let's look at how different parts of your body may respond to biological hunger, in its attempt to communicate to you it's needs for energy and nourishment and the other sensations you might experience:

- Stomach sensations: include rumbling, gurgling, gnawing, emptiness, dull pain, and aches

- Mind: inability to think clearly, concentrate or focus, headaches, dizziness, light-headedness. You may also have thoughts about food and eating, which is your body is being very clear about what you need to be focusing on and screaming at you to get up from your desk and take a lunch break!

- Mood: - you may be irritable and find yourself feeling quick to temper, impatient or apathetic. This is your body increasing the sense of urgency to eat

- Energy - feeling tired, lethargic

- Numbness - not being able to feel anything other than hunger and lethargy

- Nausea - you can feel so hungry that you feel nauseous

Remember: Whenever you experience the physical sensation of hunger, the kindest action you can take for your body is to meet the physical need for food, unconditionally and to do so before the feeling of physical hunger becomes an unpleasant or desperate one. In doing so, you'll promote a healthier relationship with food and reduce the risk of binge eating in response to intense physical hunger, to the point of physical pain or discomfort.

HUNGER AND FULLNESS SCALE

A tool I use with clients to help them assess the symptoms of their hunger and fullness, is called the Hunger and Fullness scale (next page).

This scale is referred to by medical professionals as a 'visual analogue rating', much like the pain rating scale you may have been assessed with by health care professionals.

Use the scale to think about how hunger or full you are will help you become more aware of your body's signals and cues for hunger and fullness. This scale will help you complete the daily planner pages.

	Rating	Description
Too Hungry	0	Feeling very empty. Likely to be experiencing headaches, feel faint and dizziness, stomach pains, nausea, lethargy, very low mood.
	1	'Hangry'. Feel irritable and anxious. Unable to concentrate or focus. Can't think about anything other than food.
	2	Very keen to eat a meal! Stomach rumbling and feeling empty. Thinking about food a lot.
Comfortable Range	3	Hungry and would happily eat something but there's no sense of urgency.
	4	A little bit hungry. Could use a snack or dessert. Not really thinking about food.
	5	Neutral / Neither hungry nor full
	6	Beginning to feel full.
	7	Eaten enough and now feel satisfied.
Too Full	8	A little too full. A sense of having eaten a little more than needed. Feel like I could have stopped a few bites ago. It'll be quite a while before I want to eat again.
	9	Feel physically uncomfortable and very bloated. Could use a nap (think Christmas dinner full)
	10	Feeling so full that it hurts. Feel sick. Associated with binge eating.

DAILY PLANNER: DEVELOPING BODY AWARENESS

For the next 30 days, take a few minutes each day to complete these planner pages.

Day 1	Today's Date:
Today I am feeling…	
Today I am grateful for…	
How does your body feel today? Any tension? Any pains?	
At any point today, did you allow yourself to become too hungry?	
What is something you could do today to care for your body and mind?	

Day 2	Today's Date:
Today I am feeling…	
Today I am grateful for…	
How does your body feel today? Any tension? Any pains?	
At any point today, did you allow yourself to become too hungry?	
What is something you could do today to care for your body and mind?	

Day 3	Today's Date:
Today I am feeling…	
Today I am grateful for…	
How does your body feel today? Any tension? Any pains?	
At any point today, did you allow yourself to become too hungry?	
What is something you could do today to care for your body and mind?	

Day 4	Today's Date:
Today I am feeling…	
Today I am grateful for…	
How does your body feel today? Any tension? Any pains?	
At any point today, did you allow yourself to become too hungry?	
What is something you could do today to care for your body and mind?	

Day 5	Today's Date:
Today I am feeling…	
Today I am grateful for…	
How does your body feel today? Any tension? Any pains?	
At any point today, did you allow yourself to become too hungry?	
What is something you could do today to care for your body and mind?	

Day 6	Today's Date:
Today I am feeling…	
Today I am grateful for…	
How does your body feel today? Any tension? Any pains?	
At any point today, did you allow yourself to become too hungry?	
What is something you could do today to care for your body and mind?	

Day 7	Today's Date:
Today I am feeling…	
Today I am grateful for…	
How does your body feel today? Any tension? Any pains?	
At any point today, did you allow yourself to become too hungry?	
What is something you could do today to care for your body and mind?	

Day 8	Today's Date:
Today I am feeling…	
Today I am grateful for…	
How does your body feel today? Any tension? Any pains?	
At any point today, did you allow yourself to become too hungry?	
What is something you could do today to care for your body and mind?	

Day 9	Today's Date:
Today I am feeling…	
Today I am grateful for…	
How does your body feel today? Any tension? Any pains?	
At any point today, did you allow yourself to become too hungry?	
What is something you could do today to care for your body and mind?	

Day 10	Today's Date:
Today I am feeling…	
Today I am grateful for…	
How does your body feel today? Any tension? Any pains?	
At any point today, did you allow yourself to become too hungry?	
What is something you could do today to care for your body and mind?	

Day 11	Today's Date:
Today I am feeling…	
Today I am grateful for…	
How does your body feel today? Any tension? Any pains?	
At any point today, did you allow yourself to become too hungry?	
What is something you could do today to care for your body and mind?	

Day 12	Today's Date:
Today I am feeling...	
Today I am grateful for...	
How does your body feel today? Any tension? Any pains?	
At any point today, did you allow yourself to become too hungry?	
What is something you could do today to care for your body and mind?	

Day 13	Today's Date:
Today I am feeling…	
Today I am grateful for…	
How does your body feel today? Any tension? Any pains?	
At any point today, did you allow yourself to become too hungry?	
What is something you could do today to care for your body and mind?	

Day 14	Today's Date:
Today I am feeling…	
Today I am grateful for…	
How does your body feel today? Any tension? Any pains?	
At any point today, did you allow yourself to become too hungry?	
What is something you could do today to care for your body and mind?	

Day 15	Today's Date:
Today I am feeling…	
Today I am grateful for…	
How does your body feel today? Any tension? Any pains?	
At any point today, did you allow yourself to become too hungry?	
What is something you could do today to care for your body and mind?	

Day 16	Today's Date:
Today I am feeling...	
Today I am grateful for...	
How does your body feel today? Any tension? Any pains?	
At any point today, did you allow yourself to become too hungry?	
What is something you could do today to care for your body and mind?	

Day 17	Today's Date:
Today I am feeling...	
Today I am grateful for...	
How does your body feel today? Any tension? Any pains?	
At any point today, did you allow yourself to become too hungry?	
What is something you could do today to care for your body and mind?	

Day 18	Today's Date:
Today I am feeling…	
Today I am grateful for…	
How does your body feel today? Any tension? Any pains?	
At any point today, did you allow yourself to become too hungry?	
What is something you could do today to care for your body and mind?	

Day 19	Today's Date:
Today I am feeling…	
Today I am grateful for…	
How does your body feel today? Any tension? Any pains?	
At any point today, did you allow yourself to become too hungry?	
What is something you could do today to care for your body and mind?	

Day 20	Today's Date:
Today I am feeling…	
Today I am grateful for…	
How does your body feel today? Any tension? Any pains?	
At any point today, did you allow yourself to become too hungry?	
What is something you could do today to care for your body and mind?	

Day 21	Today's Date:
Today I am feeling…	
Today I am grateful for…	
How does your body feel today? Any tension? Any pains?	
At any point today, did you allow yourself to become too hungry?	
What is something you could do today to care for your body and mind?	

Day 22	Today's Date:
Today I am feeling...	
Today I am grateful for...	
How does your body feel today? Any tension? Any pains?	
At any point today, did you allow yourself to become too hungry?	
What is something you could do today to care for your body and mind?	

Day 23	Today's Date:
Today I am feeling…	
Today I am grateful for…	
How does your body feel today? Any tension? Any pains?	
At any point today, did you allow yourself to become too hungry?	
What is something you could do today to care for your body and mind?	

Day 24	Today's Date:
Today I am feeling…	
Today I am grateful for…	
How does your body feel today? Any tension? Any pains?	
At any point today, did you allow yourself to become too hungry?	
What is something you could do today to care for your body and mind?	

Day 25	Today's Date:
Today I am feeling...	
Today I am grateful for...	
How does your body feel today? Any tension? Any pains?	
At any point today, did you allow yourself to become too hungry?	
What is something you could do today to care for your body and mind?	

Day 26	Today's Date:
Today I am feeling…	
Today I am grateful for…	
How does your body feel today? Any tension? Any pains?	
At any point today, did you allow yourself to become too hungry?	
What is something you could do today to care for your body and mind?	

Day 27	Today's Date:
Today I am feeling...	
Today I am grateful for...	
How does your body feel today? Any tension? Any pains?	
At any point today, did you allow yourself to become too hungry?	
What is something you could do today to care for your body and mind?	

Day 28	**Today's Date:**
Today I am feeling...	
Today I am grateful for...	
How does your body feel today? Any tension? Any pains?	
At any point today, did you allow yourself to become too hungry?	
What is something you could do today to care for your body and mind?	

Day 29	Today's Date:
Today I am feeling…	
Today I am grateful for…	
How does your body feel today? Any tension? Any pains?	
At any point today, did you allow yourself to become too hungry?	
What is something you could do today to care for your body and mind?	

Day 30	Today's Date:
Today I am feeling…	
Today I am grateful for…	
How does your body feel today? Any tension? Any pains?	
At any point today, did you allow yourself to become too hungry?	
What is something you could do today to care for your body and mind?	

SECTION 2: UNCONDITIONAL PERMISSION TO EAT

You are not 'good' or 'bad' based on what you eat

ASSESSING YOUR READINESS FOR EATING INTUITIVELY

Before you go further with IE, it's important to ask yourself if you're ready to implement it, or if there's still some work to do around body image and ditching diet culture.

If you find that you do still have some work left to do, this is fine! You may wish to with the free 6 day course over at:
https://www.beyondthebathroomscale.co.uk/health-mindset-starter-kit

Please answer 'yes' or 'no' to the following statements, to assess your readiness.

STATEMENT	YES	NO
I understand that dieting is harmful to my health.		
I understand how focusing on weight loss damages my relationship with food.		
I can tell the difference between physical hunger and emotional hunger.		
I can cope with my emotions without turning to food.		
I can identify my signs physical/biological hunger.		
I can tell the difference between pleasant gentle hunger and unpleasant ravenous hunger.		
I can identify my signs of fullness.		

I can tell the difference between a pleasant feeling of fullness and feeling uncomfortably stuffed.		
I can recognise when I'm hungry for a meal, vs only hungry enough for snack.		
I can experience pleasure and satisfaction from eating a meal.		

If you've ticked mostly 'yes', then you are ready to begin applying the principles of IE, which we'll be working on throughout this planner.

If you still have quite a few ticks in 'no' column, that's fine too. This process takes time and is vital that you're patient and compassionate towards yourself throughout the process.

I recommend you spend some more time reading around the topics of body positivity and Health at Every Size before you move on with IE. This ensures you have a solid foundation in which to build on and helps prevent 'relapses' into the dieting mindset.

I have lots of free resources over on Beyond The Bathroom Scale to help with exactly this, so be sure to sign up for the free 6-day course on making peace with food and your body:

https://www.beyondthebathroomscale.co.uk/health-mindset-starter-kit

IDENTIFYING YOUR FOOD FEARS AND BELIEFS

In the following exercise I want you to not down your food fears and beliefs and then analysing them and reframing them. noting down your inner voice and food fears.

To get you started, here are some examples of common food fears and beliefs:

- "I need to lose weight before I try to make peace with food. "
- "If I allow myself to eat this forbidden food, I won't stop eating it "
- "If I allow myself to eat what I truly want, I won't eat anything healthy"

Let's look at how we would analyse and then reframe each of these fears.

"I NEED TO LOSE WEIGHT BEFORE I TRY TO MAKE PEACE WITH FOOD."

Analyse it: this is an echo from diet mentality and suggests underlying boy image issues. Remember: you are practicing IE because you want to feel at ease around food and until you make peace with food, you'll continue to binge eat which is harming your health.

Reframe: focusing on weight loss has always failed me. I need to try something totally different by focusing on making peace with food by practicing IE and work on improving my body image, to improve my overall health.

"IF I ALLOW MYSELF TO EAT THIS FORBIDDEN FOOD, I WON'T STOP EATING IT"

Analyse it: having a list of forbidden or restricted food stems from dieting.

Reframe it: I only feel powerless around this food because I've restricted it for so long. the more often I give myself unconditional permission to eat it, the less power it will have over me. I'll become bored of it eventually and more aware of how the food makes me feel physically which will eventually enable me to stop eating it when I've had enough of it without feeling deprived.

"IF I ALLOW MYSELF TO EAT WHAT I TRULY WANT, I WON'T EAT ANYTHING HEALTHY"

Analyse it: when dieting I forced myself to eat foods I perceived as healthy and this made me resent these foods.

Reframe it: it's better for my overall health to make peace with food. I can focus on gentle nutrition later.

Use the food fears exercise on the next page try the belief / analysis / reframe exercise with your own food fears.

MY FOOD FEARS

BELIEF	ANALYSIS	REFRAME

FORBIDDEN FOODS & UNCONDITIONAL PERMISSION TO EAT

One of the most important aspects of IE is giving yourself unconditional permission to eat, which requires you to lose the food rules and addressing your food fears.

Unconditional permission to eat is an aspect of IE which often gets overlooked when people misinterpret IE as the 'hunger and fullness' diet. What we really don't want to be doing here is denying ourselves a certain food for whatever reason, including denying yourself a food that you want, because you're not hungry. This is where IE becomes viewed as just another diet.

I'd like you to use the forbidden foods table below. In this exercise, you will be listing the foods you've told yourself you cannot have for whatever reason.

Side note: Don't include foods you're allergic too or must avoid for health reasons, we're talking about the foods you avoid because of various food fears. Take am moment now to jot down in the table a list of foods you avoid and note down how you eat them and what impact eating them has on you.

MY (PREVIOUSLY) FORBIDDEN FOODS

FOOD	HOW DO I EAT IT? E.G. QUICKLY, RUSHED, URGENTLY, OR SLOW AND MINDFULLY.	HOW DOES EATING IT MAKE ME FEEL? DOES IT AFFECT HOW I EAT FOR THE REST OF THE DAY? HOW DOES IT MAKE ME FEEL?

INCREASING THE FAMILIARITY OF FORBIDDEN FOODS

What I'd like you to do over the next few days, weeks or even months, depending on how many foods you have your list, is to give yourself permission to eat some of these foods at some point and then keep eating these same foods over and over again.

What we're aiming for here, is to lessen the enticement of the food, and eliminate any feelings of guilt you may have for eating it, by increasing its familiarity.

I'm going to give you a personal example now from my own experience of IE. Before I started practicing IE, I had developed frequent cravings for a dish on a pub menu, a pub I often went to with my son for dinner in the week. This dish was a curry banquet, with lots of sides - chips, rice, onion bhajis, naan bread - the lot!

For months before I came across IE, I used to chastise myself for wanting it, ordering it, and eating it. The fear of calories and gaining weight stifled my enjoyment of it and made me feel guilt instead of satisfaction. I'd eat it fast and then I'd feel really bloated afterwards.

For the first few months of starting IE, I gave myself unconditional permission to order it anyway and enjoy it without judgment and it was the *only* thing I ever ordered each week, sometimes twice a week, for a few months.

Eventually I became so familiar with it, that I got bored of it even though I still enjoyed its taste. I had stopped feel guilty when I ate it, and my desire for it lessened. Instead I fancied a nice steak which didn't leave me feeling bloated, or some fish and chips if I felt particularly hungry that day.

When I choose what I want for dinner nowadays, I choose based on my hunger levels and what I genuinely fancy eating. Now that my 'forbidden foods' are so familiar to me, they've lost their allure and because I'm so relaxed around these foods now, I now have the mental space to be more conscious of how I physically feel while eating them. Sometimes I'm just not hungry enough for such a big meal, and that's ok, because I know I can order it any other time I want it, with zero feelings of deprivation, denial, or guilt.

Try this approach with your forbidden foods list, become familiar with them over the next few weeks or months and notice how your feelings towards these foods shift. You can use the next 30 days of planner to record your thoughts.

DAILY PLANNER: UNCONDITIONAL PERMISSION TO EAT

For the next 30 days, take a few minutes each day to complete these planner pages.

Tip: Use the Hunger & Fullness Scale to help

Day 1	Today's Date:
Today I am feeling…	
Today I am grateful for…	
Did I give myself unconditional permission to eat?	
Did I remain aware of my hunger and fullness cues?	
What happened? How did I feel afterwards? Did I take time to savour it? Was it a pleasurable experience?	

Day 2	Today's Date:
Today I am feeling…	
Today I am grateful for…	
Did I give myself unconditional permission to eat?	
Did I remain aware of my hunger and fullness cues?	
What happened? How did I feel afterwards? Did I take time to savour it? Was it a pleasurable experience?	

Day 3	Today's Date:
Today I am feeling…	
Today I am grateful for…	
Did I give myself unconditional permission to eat?	
Did I remain aware of my hunger and fullness cues?	
What happened? How did I feel afterwards? Did I take time to savour it? Was it a pleasurable experience?	

Day 4	Today's Date:
Today I am feeling…	
Today I am grateful for…	
Did I give myself unconditional permission to eat?	
Did I remain aware of my hunger and fullness cues?	
What happened? How did I feel afterwards? Did I take time to savour it? Was it a pleasurable experience?	

Day 5	Today's Date:
Today I am feeling…	
Today I am grateful for…	
Did I give myself unconditional permission to eat?	
Did I remain aware of my hunger and fullness cues?	
What happened? How did I feel afterwards? Did I take time to savour it? Was it a pleasurable experience?	

Day 6	Today's Date:
Today I am feeling...	
Today I am grateful for...	
Did I give myself unconditional permission to eat?	
Did I remain aware of my hunger and fullness cues?	
What happened? How did I feel afterwards? Did I take time to savour it? Was it a pleasurable experience?	

Day 7	Today's Date:
Today I am feeling…	
Today I am grateful for…	
Did I give myself unconditional permission to eat?	
Did I remain aware of my hunger and fullness cues?	
What happened? How did I feel afterwards? Did I take time to savour it? Was it a pleasurable experience?	

Day 8	Today's Date:
Today I am feeling…	
Today I am grateful for…	
Did I give myself unconditional permission to eat?	
Did I remain aware of my hunger and fullness cues?	
What happened? How did I feel afterwards? Did I take time to savour it? Was it a pleasurable experience?	

Day 8	Today's Date:
Today I am feeling…	
Today I am grateful for…	
Did I give myself unconditional permission to eat?	
Did I remain aware of my hunger and fullness cues?	
What happened? How did I feel afterwards? Did I take time to savour it? Was it a pleasurable experience?	

Day 9	Today's Date:
Today I am feeling…	
Today I am grateful for…	
Did I give myself unconditional permission to eat?	
Did I remain aware of my hunger and fullness cues?	
What happened? How did I feel afterwards? Did I take time to savour it? Was it a pleasurable experience?	

Day 10	Today's Date:
Today I am feeling…	
Today I am grateful for…	
Did I give myself unconditional permission to eat?	
Did I remain aware of my hunger and fullness cues?	
What happened? How did I feel afterwards? Did I take time to savour it? Was it a pleasurable experience?	

Day 11	Today's Date:
Today I am feeling…	
Today I am grateful for…	
Did I give myself unconditional permission to eat?	
Did I remain aware of my hunger and fullness cues?	
What happened? How did I feel afterwards? Did I take time to savour it? Was it a pleasurable experience?	

Day 12	Today's Date:
Today I am feeling…	
Today I am grateful for…	
Did I give myself unconditional permission to eat?	
Did I remain aware of my hunger and fullness cues?	
What happened? How did I feel afterwards? Did I take time to savour it? Was it a pleasurable experience?	

Day 13	Today's Date:
Today I am feeling…	
Today I am grateful for…	
Did I give myself unconditional permission to eat?	
Did I remain aware of my hunger and fullness cues?	
What happened? How did I feel afterwards? Did I take time to savour it? Was it a pleasurable experience?	

Day 14	Today's Date:
Today I am feeling…	
Today I am grateful for…	
Did I give myself unconditional permission to eat?	
Did I remain aware of my hunger and fullness cues?	
What happened? How did I feel afterwards? Did I take time to savour it? Was it a pleasurable experience?	

Day 15	Today's Date:
Today I am feeling…	
Today I am grateful for…	
Did I give myself unconditional permission to eat?	
Did I remain aware of my hunger and fullness cues?	
What happened? How did I feel afterwards? Did I take time to savour it? Was it a pleasurable experience?	

Day 16	Today's Date:
Today I am feeling…	
Today I am grateful for…	
Did I give myself unconditional permission to eat?	
Did I remain aware of my hunger and fullness cues?	
What happened? How did I feel afterwards? Did I take time to savour it? Was it a pleasurable experience?	

Day 17	Today's Date:
Today I am feeling…	
Today I am grateful for…	
Did I give myself unconditional permission to eat?	
Did I remain aware of my hunger and fullness cues?	
What happened? How did I feel afterwards? Did I take time to savour it? Was it a pleasurable experience?	

Day 18	Today's Date:
Today I am feeling…	
Today I am grateful for…	
Did I give myself unconditional permission to eat?	
Did I remain aware of my hunger and fullness cues?	
What happened? How did I feel afterwards? Did I take time to savour it? Was it a pleasurable experience?	

Day 19	Today's Date:
Today I am feeling…	
Today I am grateful for…	
Did I give myself unconditional permission to eat?	
Did I remain aware of my hunger and fullness cues?	
What happened? How did I feel afterwards? Did I take time to savour it? Was it a pleasurable experience?	

Day 20	Today's Date:
Today I am feeling…	
Today I am grateful for…	
Did I give myself unconditional permission to eat?	
Did I remain aware of my hunger and fullness cues?	
What happened? How did I feel afterwards? Did I take time to savour it? Was it a pleasurable experience?	

Day 21	Today's Date:
Today I am feeling…	
Today I am grateful for…	
Did I give myself unconditional permission to eat?	
Did I remain aware of my hunger and fullness cues?	
What happened? How did I feel afterwards? Did I take time to savour it? Was it a pleasurable experience?	

Day 22	**Today's Date:**
Today I am feeling...	
Today I am grateful for...	
Did I give myself unconditional permission to eat?	
Did I remain aware of my hunger and fullness cues?	
What happened? How did I feel afterwards? Did I take time to savour it? Was it a pleasurable experience?	

Day 23	**Today's Date:**
Today I am feeling…	
Today I am grateful for…	
Did I give myself unconditional permission to eat?	
Did I remain aware of my hunger and fullness cues?	
What happened? How did I feel afterwards? Did I take time to savour it? Was it a pleasurable experience?	

Day 24	Today's Date:
Today I am feeling…	
Today I am grateful for…	
Did I give myself unconditional permission to eat?	
Did I remain aware of my hunger and fullness cues?	
What happened? How did I feel afterwards? Did I take time to savour it? Was it a pleasurable experience?	

Day 25	Today's Date:
Today I am feeling…	
Today I am grateful for…	
Did I give myself unconditional permission to eat?	
Did I remain aware of my hunger and fullness cues?	
What happened? How did I feel afterwards? Did I take time to savour it? Was it a pleasurable experience?	

Day 26	Today's Date:
Today I am feeling…	
Today I am grateful for…	
Did I give myself unconditional permission to eat?	
Did I remain aware of my hunger and fullness cues?	
What happened? How did I feel afterwards? Did I take time to savour it? Was it a pleasurable experience?	

Day 27	Today's Date:
Today I am feeling…	
Today I am grateful for…	
Did I give myself unconditional permission to eat?	
Did I remain aware of my hunger and fullness cues?	
What happened? How did I feel afterwards? Did I take time to savour it? Was it a pleasurable experience?	

Day 28	Today's Date:
Today I am feeling…	
Today I am grateful for…	
Did I give myself unconditional permission to eat?	
Did I remain aware of my hunger and fullness cues?	
What happened? How did I feel afterwards? Did I take time to savour it? Was it a pleasurable experience?	

Day 29	Today's Date:
Today I am feeling…	
Today I am grateful for…	
Did I give myself unconditional permission to eat?	
Did I remain aware of my hunger and fullness cues?	
What happened? How did I feel afterwards? Did I take time to savour it? Was it a pleasurable experience?	

Day 30	Today's Date:
Today I am feeling…	
Today I am grateful for…	
Did I give myself unconditional permission to eat?	
Did I remain aware of my hunger and fullness cues?	
What happened? How did I feel afterwards? Did I take time to savour it? Was it a pleasurable experience?	

SECTION 3: MINDFUL EATING

Never eat anything you don't enjoy and truly enjoy everything you eat

WHAT IS MINDFUL EATING?

In this part, we're going to run through an enjoyable mindful eating exercise, to give you an idea of how it feels to slow down, savour and relax with your food while you're eating. This relaxed and mindful approach to eating is a key part of intuitive eating.

Eating mindfully is something a lot of us struggle with. Often, we eat in front of the tv, while on the go, or sat at our desks at work checking email. When we're not paying much attention to our food, we may find that before we know it, we've finished our food without giving a second thought to the taste, texture, or aroma of the food or how full we're feeling. In doing this, we've denied ourselves the opportunity to really immerse ourselves in the pleasurable experience of eating, leaving us still feeling like we're still lacking something after our meal.

By eating free of distractions, and while in a relaxed mindset, this frees up your mind up to focus on the pleasure you're getting from food and the physical sensations of hunger and fullness, enabling you to recognize when you're satisfied and finished eating (even if this means leaving food on the plate, or saving some for later!).

MINDFUL EATING EXERCISE

For this exercise I would like you to choose a piece of food to practice the mindful eating exercise with. Eventually, you will be able to do this with a meal, but for now I would like you to choose a single item of food. This might be square of nice chocolate or a piece of fruit. Choose something you really enjoy eating to make this the most pleasurable experience possible.

Before we begin the exercise, I'd like to set up your environment, ready for relaxed eating. This might sound a little strange or perhaps frivolous but the reason for this is that it's so important is that you feel relaxed and at ease while you're eating. You'll likely find it much easier at first, to do this at a time when you can eat alone, so no children, pets, or adults around to distract you or evoke strong emotional responses.

If possible, sit at a table (not a desk at work) or at the very least somewhere quiet and free of distractions. Switch your phone to 'do not disturb', turn off any screens and avoid background noise like music or people talking.

- Begin by placing your chosen food on a plate, napkin or in its packaging in front of you.

- For a moment I would like you to close your eyes and take a deep breath in through your nose, hold it and take a deep breath out through your mouth. Repeat this a few times until you feel calm and relaxed.

- Now take a moment to check in with how you're feeling emotionally, while continuing to breathe deeply until you feel calm and relaxed. We are not going to rush through this experience, we are going to savour each moment by engaging all our senses.

- Now open your eyes and look at the food in front of you. Visually inspect the food like it's new to you. Observe the colour, shape, and texture of the food. Is it rough or smooth? If you're struggling with this, imagine you're describing the food to someone who has never seen it.

- Next, lean in to gently smell the food. Does it have an aroma? Is it strong or subtle? How would you describe the scent to another person?

- Now pick up the food and hold it, or if you have a meal in front of you, begin to cut into it or place some on your fork or spoon. If you're holding it, notice how it feels in your hand. Is it rough or smooth? Sticky, crumbly, soft, hard, heavy, or light? If you're using utensils, how easy was it to cut the food or place it on your fork or spoon - is it tough to cut through? or easy to pick up with the utensil?

- Take a small bite of your food, does it make a sound when you take a bite? Does it snap or crunch? Is it slurpy or is it quiet, almost soundless? With the food in your mouth, resist swallowing it right away.

- Gently roll the food around in your mouth and observe how it feels in your mouth. Is it warm or cold? What is the texture of the food, is it liquid and easy to swallow, solid and requires chewing? Does it change while it's on your tongue? Getting soggy, breaking apart or perhaps melting?

- How does it taste? Sweet, sour, bitter, salty? Is it bland or strong? Does the taste change as it sits on your tongue? Is there a range or mix of different flavours or is it uniform?

- Next chew your food and swallow it when you feel ready. As you continue eating with care and your full attention, you may like to give thought to the origins and journey of your food. Where has it come from? Has it been manufactured, grown or reared? Who has been involved in the process of getting the food from its origins to your plate? Take a moment to feel gratitude for the food and its journey.

How did it feel to complete this exercise? Use the space below to reflect:

STOPPING WHEN FULL

We're now going to take IE one step further, by practicing stopping eating when we feel full. What's important at this stage (and makes all the difference between this being about mindfulness rather than another form of a diet) is to ask yourself, does this idea of stopping eating when you feel full, seem difficult? If so, please don't attempt to implement this just yet. Instead, you need to reflect have you really made peace with food at this stage. It's ok if you haven't, this can take a long time to come around to.

If you sense you're struggling to stop eating when you're full, continue working on analysing your fears around food, and your beliefs about weight and food rules. Keep exposing yourself to your 'forbidden foods' until you no longer feel guilt for eating them or feel cravings towards them (experiencing either of these is a sign you're still restricting the food on some level, perhaps psychologically).

Let's also look at other factors which prevent you from stopping when you're full. For example, some of us have a strong need to clear our plates, regardless of hunger cues, and others simply can't bring themselves to refuse or waste food that's on offer.

CLEAN PLATE MENTALITY - A VALUE OR HABIT?

If you suspect that the need to clean your plate, regardless of your fullness level, *is* a habit, then work on slowing down your eating by practicing the mindful eating exercise more often and taking time to pause, put down utensils and ask yourself:

- Do I still feel hungry?
- Am I still getting pleasure from this food?
- How do I feel physically now?

- Am I feeling full?

If it's about values and not wanting to leave food, waste it or look impolite, then consider taking leftovers with you to eat later in the day or with a meal the next day.

LEARNING HOW TO POLITELY REFUSE FOOD

Are you someone who struggles to turn down the offer of extra food when you know you're already feeling full? In some situations, the offer of more food is just a case of being accommodating. After all, no host or restaurant wants someone to leave feeling hungry or dissatisfied!

In other situations, you may get a sense that the other person gains pleasure from seeing you eat. Sometimes, people use food as a way of expressing love or care.

If this is a case, reflect on whether you're only eating to please this person, to make them happy or to avoid offending them. The trouble with this people-pleasing attitude, is it's harming your health, both emotionally (feeling like your feelings take lower priority) and physically (making you feel uncomfortably full).

Take a moment to reflect on using the space on the next page why you struggle to refuse food.

- Is it a fear of upsetting or offending others?
- Or is it a case of not wanting to turn down extra food because of the fear of scarcity (I might not get to eat this again)?

WHY DO YOU THINK YOU STRUGGLE TO REFUSE FOOD WHEN YOU'RE ALREADY FULL?

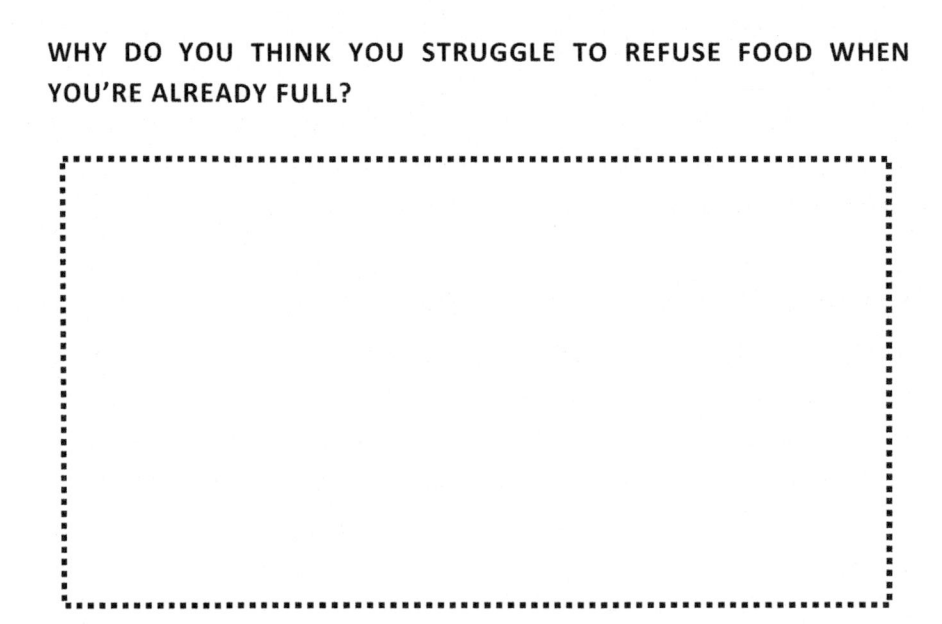

Next, try thinking of and rehearsing some simple statements for politely declining food in different circumstances.

Here are some examples:

- "No thank you" (remember no is a complete sentence)

- "It looks amazing, but I really couldn't possibly fit anything else in, I'm feeling pleasantly full after that delicious meal."

- "I'm so sorry, I've just eaten and didn't know you'd be serving food. It all looks delicious but I'm too full to try any right now. I wouldn't want to think of your effort and food going to waste, so I'm happy to take some home with me if you have too many leftovers."

Take a moment now to jot down in the space on the next page, some responses that feel right for you in the situations you often find yourself in.

SENTENCES I CAN SAY WHEN I WANT TO POLITELY DECLINE FOOD:

HANDLING WEIGHT GAIN & THE URGE TO DIET

In this exercise I'm going to outline the steps I want you to take if at any point you panic about weight gain and feel tempted to start a diet.

To begin with, I want you to take a moment to reflect on what triggered you to want to start a diet or weigh yourself.

- What happened?
- What was your thought response?
- How are you feeling emotionally?

Try to unpick where these thoughts and emotions have come from. If you struggle with this, imagine it's your friend coming to you with this problem and you're advising them.

Here's an example:

EVENT: A friend has asked me to be a bridesmaid

THOUGHT RESPONSE:

I'll have to be measured for a dress! All my old friends and possibly my ex will see me! I need to look hot. I should start a diet to lose weight before the wedding!

EMOTIONS: Nervous, anxious, scared, a little bit excited.

UNPICKING THESE THOUGHTS AND EMOTIONS:

I'm worried that my friends and ex will judge me for my weight.

TALK YOURSELF DOWN:

Only the tailor at the shop needs to know my dress size! Who cares? Everyone else will be worrying about what they look like! My old friends will be glad to see me and have a chance to catch up.

Being confident and happy is sexy, and I have lots of personal accomplishments to talk about when asked, such as my new job and side project.

Try the dieting Triggers Exercise on the next page.

DIETING TRIGGERS EXERCISE

WHAT HAPPENED?

WHAT WAS YOUR INITIAL THOUGHT RESPONSE?

HOW DID THIS MAKE YOU FEEL?

TRY TO UNPICK WHERE THESE THOUGHTS AND EMOTIONS CAME FROM.

TALK YOURSELF DOWN FROM THE DIETING LEDGE (USE THE STEPS LISTED BELOW TO HELP):

```
..................................................................
:                                                                :
:                                                                :
:                                                                :
:                                                                :
:                                                                :
:                                                                :
:                                                                :
:                                                                :
:                                                                :
:                                                                :
:                                                                :
..................................................................
```

STEPS TO TAKE TO HANDLE DIET TRIGGERS

1. Look at body positive social media - make your account a safe online space to retreat to
2. Remind yourself of your dieting history and that diets haven't worked in the past: Have you ever managed to keep weight of for a few years or more? Did losing weight ever stop you from feel obsessed with food, exercise, and the scale? Did a diet ever raise your self-confidence, improve your sense of worth and make you feel good about your body, or did you feel like your body can always be improved in some way?
3. Read books and listen to podcasts by dietitians who speak about the failings of the diet industry and the benefits of intuitive eating
4. Join IE Facebook groups to seek support from other people going through the same struggles as you

If you put all these strategies in place, you'll be able to talk yourself down from the dieting ledge and find yourself able to continue with the amazing progress you're making when it comes to practicing intuitive eating.

DAILY PLANNER: MINDFUL EATING

For the next 30 days, take a few minutes each day to complete these planner pages.

Day 1	Today's Date:
Today I am feeling…	
Today I am grateful for…	
Did you eat at least one meal or snack today, without distraction? Did you enjoy it?	
Which foods kept you feeling full for longer today? Why do you think this was?	
Did you feel hungry in time for your next meal? If not, why do you think this was?	

Day 2	Today's Date:
Today I am feeling…	
Today I am grateful for…	
Did you eat at least one meal or snack today, without distraction? Did you enjoy it?	
Which foods kept you feeling full for longer today? Why do you think this was?	
Did you feel hungry in time for your next meal? If not, why do you think this was?	

Day 3	Today's Date:
Today I am feeling…	
Today I am grateful for…	
Did you eat at least one meal or snack today, without distraction? Did you enjoy it?	
Which foods kept you feeling full for longer today? Why do you think this was?	
Did you feel hungry in time for your next meal? If not, why do you think this was?	

Day 4	Today's Date:
Today I am feeling…	
Today I am grateful for…	
Did you eat at least one meal or snack today, without distraction? Did you enjoy it?	
Which foods kept you feeling full for longer today? Why do you think this was?	
Did you feel hungry in time for your next meal? If not, why do you think this was?	

Day 5	Today's Date:
Today I am feeling…	
Today I am grateful for…	
Did you eat at least one meal or snack today, without distraction? Did you enjoy it?	
Which foods kept you feeling full for longer today? Why do you think this was?	
Did you feel hungry in time for your next meal? If not, why do you think this was?	

Day 6	Today's Date:
Today I am feeling…	
Today I am grateful for…	
Did you eat at least one meal or snack today, without distraction? Did you enjoy it?	
Which foods kept you feeling full for longer today? Why do you think this was?	
Did you feel hungry in time for your next meal? If not, why do you think this was?	

Day 7	Today's Date:
Today I am feeling…	
Today I am grateful for…	
Did you eat at least one meal or snack today, without distraction? Did you enjoy it?	
Which foods kept you feeling full for longer today? Why do you think this was?	
Did you feel hungry in time for your next meal? If not, why do you think this was?	

Day 8	Today's Date:
Today I am feeling…	
Today I am grateful for…	
Did you eat at least one meal or snack today, without distraction? Did you enjoy it?	
Which foods kept you feeling full for longer today? Why do you think this was?	
Did you feel hungry in time for your next meal? If not, why do you think this was?	

Day 9	Today's Date:
Today I am feeling…	
Today I am grateful for…	
Did you eat at least one meal or snack today, without distraction? Did you enjoy it?	
Which foods kept you feeling full for longer today? Why do you think this was?	
Did you feel hungry in time for your next meal? If not, why do you think this was?	

Day 10	**Today's Date:**
Today I am feeling…	
Today I am grateful for…	
Did you eat at least one meal or snack today, without distraction? Did you enjoy it?	
Which foods kept you feeling full for longer today? Why do you think this was?	
Did you feel hungry in time for your next meal? If not, why do you think this was?	

Day 11	Today's Date:
Today I am feeling…	
Today I am grateful for…	
Did you eat at least one meal or snack today, without distraction? Did you enjoy it?	
Which foods kept you feeling full for longer today? Why do you think this was?	
Did you feel hungry in time for your next meal? If not, why do you think this was?	

Day 12	Today's Date:
Today I am feeling…	
Today I am grateful for…	
Did you eat at least one meal or snack today, without distraction? Did you enjoy it?	
Which foods kept you feeling full for longer today? Why do you think this was?	
Did you feel hungry in time for your next meal? If not, why do you think this was?	

Day 13	Today's Date:
Today I am feeling…	
Today I am grateful for…	
Did you eat at least one meal or snack today, without distraction? Did you enjoy it?	
Which foods kept you feeling full for longer today? Why do you think this was?	
Did you feel hungry in time for your next meal? If not, why do you think this was?	

Day 14	Today's Date:
Today I am feeling…	
Today I am grateful for…	
Did you eat at least one meal or snack today, without distraction? Did you enjoy it?	
Which foods kept you feeling full for longer today? Why do you think this was?	
Did you feel hungry in time for your next meal? If not, why do you think this was?	

Day 15	Today's Date:
Today I am feeling…	
Today I am grateful for…	
Did you eat at least one meal or snack today, without distraction? Did you enjoy it?	
Which foods kept you feeling full for longer today? Why do you think this was?	
Did you feel hungry in time for your next meal? If not, why do you think this was?	

Day 16	Today's Date:
Today I am feeling...	
Today I am grateful for...	
Did you eat at least one meal or snack today, without distraction? Did you enjoy it?	
Which foods kept you feeling full for longer today? Why do you think this was?	
Did you feel hungry in time for your next meal? If not, why do you think this was?	

Day 17	Today's Date:
Today I am feeling…	
Today I am grateful for…	
Did you eat at least one meal or snack today, without distraction? Did you enjoy it?	
Which foods kept you feeling full for longer today? Why do you think this was?	
Did you feel hungry in time for your next meal? If not, why do you think this was?	

Day 18	Today's Date:
Today I am feeling...	
Today I am grateful for...	
Did you eat at least one meal or snack today, without distraction? Did you enjoy it?	
Which foods kept you feeling full for longer today? Why do you think this was?	
Did you feel hungry in time for your next meal? If not, why do you think this was?	

Day 19	**Today's Date:**
Today I am feeling…	
Today I am grateful for…	
Did you eat at least one meal or snack today, without distraction? Did you enjoy it?	
Which foods kept you feeling full for longer today? Why do you think this was?	
Did you feel hungry in time for your next meal? If not, why do you think this was?	

Day 20	Today's Date:
Today I am feeling…	
Today I am grateful for…	
Did you eat at least one meal or snack today, without distraction? Did you enjoy it?	
Which foods kept you feeling full for longer today? Why do you think this was?	
Did you feel hungry in time for your next meal? If not, why do you think this was?	

Day 21	**Today's Date:**
Today I am feeling…	
Today I am grateful for…	
Did you eat at least one meal or snack today, without distraction? Did you enjoy it?	
Which foods kept you feeling full for longer today? Why do you think this was?	
Did you feel hungry in time for your next meal? If not, why do you think this was?	

Day 22	Today's Date:
Today I am feeling…	
Today I am grateful for…	
Did you eat at least one meal or snack today, without distraction? Did you enjoy it?	
Which foods kept you feeling full for longer today? Why do you think this was?	
Did you feel hungry in time for your next meal? If not, why do you think this was?	

Day 23	Today's Date:
Today I am feeling…	
Today I am grateful for…	
Did you eat at least one meal or snack today, without distraction? Did you enjoy it?	
Which foods kept you feeling full for longer today? Why do you think this was?	
Did you feel hungry in time for your next meal? If not, why do you think this was?	

Day 24	**Today's Date:**
Today I am feeling…	
Today I am grateful for…	
Did you eat at least one meal or snack today, without distraction? Did you enjoy it?	
Which foods kept you feeling full for longer today? Why do you think this was?	
Did you feel hungry in time for your next meal? If not, why do you think this was?	

Day 25	**Today's Date:**
Today I am feeling…	
Today I am grateful for…	
Did you eat at least one meal or snack today, without distraction? Did you enjoy it?	
Which foods kept you feeling full for longer today? Why do you think this was?	
Did you feel hungry in time for your next meal? If not, why do you think this was?	

Day 26	Today's Date:
Today I am feeling...	
Today I am grateful for...	
Did you eat at least one meal or snack today, without distraction? Did you enjoy it?	
Which foods kept you feeling full for longer today? Why do you think this was?	
Did you feel hungry in time for your next meal? If not, why do you think this was?	

Day 27	Today's Date:
Today I am feeling…	
Today I am grateful for…	
Did you eat at least one meal or snack today, without distraction? Did you enjoy it?	
Which foods kept you feeling full for longer today? Why do you think this was?	
Did you feel hungry in time for your next meal? If not, why do you think this was?	

Day 28	Today's Date:
Today I am feeling…	
Today I am grateful for…	
Did you eat at least one meal or snack today, without distraction? Did you enjoy it?	
Which foods kept you feeling full for longer today? Why do you think this was?	
Did you feel hungry in time for your next meal? If not, why do you think this was?	

Day 29	Today's Date:
Today I am feeling…	
Today I am grateful for…	
Did you eat at least one meal or snack today, without distraction? Did you enjoy it?	
Which foods kept you feeling full for longer today? Why do you think this was?	
Did you feel hungry in time for your next meal? If not, why do you think this was?	

Day 30	Today's Date:
Today I am feeling…	
Today I am grateful for…	
Did you eat at least one meal or snack today, without distraction? Did you enjoy it?	
Which foods kept you feeling full for longer today? Why do you think this was?	
Did you feel hungry in time for your next meal? If not, why do you think this was?	

END OF PLANNER REFLECTIONS

Like any relationship, the one you have with food and your body, requires trust and gentle compassion.

PEACEFUL EATING SELF-ASSESSMENT REVISITED

Let's see how much progress you've made with developing a peaceful relationship with food. Read through the statements below and tick the ones you agree with or feel apply to you most of the time.

I avoid certain foods groups or ingredients (which I do not have an allergy or intolerance to) because I believe that cutting these foods out will help with weight loss. (e.g. carbs, grains, gluten, dairy).	
I permit myself to have 'cheat days' or 'cheat meals', where I allow myself to eat whatever I want.	
If I want to eat something I view as 'extra' in a day, like a dessert, I feel like I need to exercise more, i.e. the 'burn it to earn it' philosophy.	
If I know I'm going out for a meal with friends in the evening, I cut back on food in the day to account for it.	
I carefully eat all week, and then eat whatever I want at the weekends, regardless of how hungry or full I feel.	
I count and track calories.	

I try to adhere to a calorie or points/Syns goal most days, regardless of how hungry or full I am.	
If I eat 'forbidden' foods ('treats', 'junk' or 'bad'), I feel like I've blown it and then experience the 'f*ck it effect', where I eat everything in large quantities and ignore my hunger/fullness cues.	
If I feel like I ate too much at one meal, I deliberately eat less at the next to 'make up for it', regardless of how hungry I am.	
I describe my day of food as either 'good' or 'bad'.	
I say things like "getting back on plan" or "falling off the wagon".	
I eat foods I don't like because I consider them 'healthy'.	
I have a list of foods I consider 'bad' or 'forbidden'.	

I refer to some foods as 'guilt free'.	
When I feel hungry, I look for ways to distract myself from the urge to eat.	
I feel the need to clear my plate, regardless of how full I feel.	
I struggle to recognise fullness long before I feel uncomfortably full	
I have difficulty judging how much to eat.	
I have difficulty deciding what I should eat.	
I decide what and how much to eat based on my calorie (or points/Syns) goal for the day, regardless of how hungry I'm feeling.	

Tally up the number of ticks and make a note of your score below. Compare this score to the score you've written down at the start of the planner to see how far you've progressed.

Today's date	
My score	

FINAL REFLECTIONS

Now that you've completed this workbook, take some time to reflect on what you've learned, using the prompts below and jot your thoughts down using the space on the next page.

- How do you feel after giving yourself unconditional permission to eat foods you've previously restricted?

- How did it feel to practise the mindful eating exercise?

- Which foods did you find filled you up for the longest?

- Do you feel like you will be able to handle the urge to diet in future?

WHERE TO GO FROM HERE?

Congratulations on completing *the 90 Day Peaceful Eating Planner*!

Remember, your recovery doesn't end here and will be an ongoing process. Do you feel like you would benefit from more information, cognitive behavioural therapy exercises, helpful resources, and monthly support?

In *the Health Mindset Programme*™, we cover the topics of Diet Culture, Intuitive Eating, Emotional Eating and Body Positivity, in depth and in short, to-the-point, actionable video-based lessons. There's also workbooks and guides to support you in healing the relationship you have with food, exercise, and your body.

The online programme is self-paced and spaced out over 6-7 months, so you can dip in and out of it whenever you have the time. It is designed to be a safe, informative, and healing environment to enable you to recover from a lifetime of dieting and disordered eating.

It's time to make peace with food and your body and become healthy, confident, and happy.

Find out more about the 6-month online programme and join here: **https://www.beyondthebathroomscale.co.uk/thehealthmindsetprogramme/**

If you haven't already, you can sign up for the free six-day taster course here: **https://www.beyondthebathroomscale.co.uk/health-mindset-starter-kit**

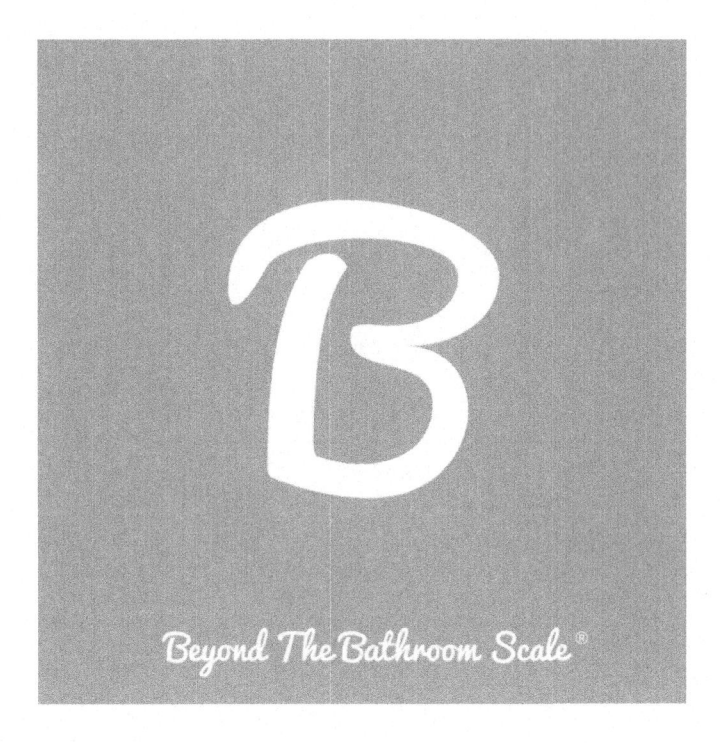

Follow on Facebook and Instagram: @Beyondthebathroomscale